Dysautonomia signs

Full informative guide on how dysautonomia affect and regulate bodily functions such as heart rate

Dr Joe smith

Contents

chapter1...3

introduction to dysautonomia
treatment 3

chapter2...18

dysautonomia diagnosis 18

chapter3...25

dysautonomia nhs 25

chapter4...32

dysautonomia signs 32

The end 38

chapter1

introduction to dysautonomia treatment

Dysautonomia is a complex and often debilitating condition that affects millions of people worldwide. It is a disorder of the autonomic nervous system, which regulates important bodily functions such as heart rate, blood pressure, digestion, and temperature control. When this system malfunctions, it can lead to a wide range of uncomfortable and sometimes life-threatening symptoms. Unfortunately, there is currently no cure for dysautonomia, and treatment options focus on managing and alleviating symptoms. However, with the right approach, many people living with dysautonomia can find relief and improve their quality of life. In this article, we will explore the different treatment options available for those with dysautonomia and discuss some strategies for managing the condition successfully. Medications Medications are often used to manage the symptoms of dysautonomia. There is no one-size-fits-all approach when it comes to treatment, and different medications may be prescribed depending on the type of dysautonomia and the individual's specific symptoms. Some common medications used to treat dysautonomia include: 1. Beta blockers - These drugs are used to lower blood pressure, heart rate, and anxiety. They work by blocking the effects of adrenaline, a hormone that can cause an increase in heart rate, blood pressure, and other symptoms of dysautonomia. 2. Fludrocortisone - This medication is a synthetic form of aldosterone, a hormone that helps regulate fluid and electrolyte balance in the body. Fludrocortisone can be helpful in managing hypotension (low blood pressure) and other symptoms of dysautonomia. 3. Midodrine - This drug is used to treat orthostatic hypotension, a drop in blood pressure that occurs when standing up. Midodrine works by causing the blood vessels to narrow, which helps to raise blood pressure. 4. Antidepressants - Some antidepressant medications, like selective serotonin reuptake inhibitors (SSRIs) and serotonin-norepinephrine reuptake inhibitors (SNRIs), may be prescribed to manage dysautonomia symptoms such as depression, anxiety, and fatigue. While these medications can be effective in managing dysautonomia symptoms, they may also cause side effects, which can be challenging to manage for some individuals. Therefore, it is essential to work closely with a healthcare provider to find the right medication and dosage that works best for each person. Lifestyle Changes In addition to medication, lifestyle changes can play a crucial role in managing dysautonomia symptoms. Here are a few tips to consider: 1. Stay hydrated - Dehydration can worsen symptoms of dysautonomia, so it is important to drink plenty of water and electrolyte beverages throughout the day. It's best to avoid sugary drinks and caffeine, as they can cause dehydration and may trigger symptoms. 2. Avoid triggers - Certain foods, environmental factors, and physical activities can trigger or worsen symptoms of dysautonomia. By identifying and avoiding these triggers, individuals may be able to better manage their condition. It's essential to keep a journal to track symptoms and identify potential triggers. 3. Use compression garments - Compression garments, such as compression stockings or full-body suits, can help improve circulation and reduce blood pooling in the legs. They can be especially useful for individuals with orthostatic hypotension. 4. Exercise regularly - While excessive physical activity can worsen dysautonomia symptoms, gentle and regular exercise can help improve cardiovascular fitness and circulation. Exercise can also reduce anxiety and stress, which are common comorbidities of dysautonomia. Alternative Therapies Some individuals with dysautonomia may find relief from alternative therapies, such as acupuncture, massage, and chiropractic care. These treatments can help reduce muscle tension, improve circulation, and promote relaxation, which may alleviate symptoms. Furthermore, mind-body practices, such as yoga, tai chi, and meditation, may also be beneficial. These practices can help manage stress and anxiety, improve sleep quality, and boost overall well-being. Invasive Procedures In severe cases of dysautonomia where symptoms are unmanageable with medications and lifestyle changes, invasive procedures may be considered. One example is a pacemaker, which can be implanted to help regulate heart rate and blood pressure. Other invasive approaches include spinal cord stimulation and vagus nerve stimulation, which may also help manage symptoms. Managing Dysautonomia holistically While medications and lifestyle changes can help manage the symptoms of dysautonomia, there is increasing evidence that managing the condition holistically can lead to better outcomes. This approach involves addressing not only physical symptoms but also psychological and emotional factors that contribute to dysautonomia. For example, stress, anxiety, and depression are common comorbidities of dysautonomia and can significantly impact one's quality of life. Therefore, it is vital to manage mental health and seek support when needed. This can include therapy, support groups, and self-care practices such as mindfulness and relaxation techniques. Furthermore, a balanced and healthy diet can play a significant role in managing dysautonomia symptoms. Some people with dysautonomia may benefit from a low-carbohydrate diet, which can help regulate blood pressure and improve symptoms such as brain fog and fatigue.

Conclusion In conclusion, while there is no cure for dysautonomia, there are various treatment options available that can help manage the condition and improve quality of life. These include medications, lifestyle changes, alternative therapies, invasive procedures, and a holistic approach. Each person with dysautonomia may require a unique combination of treatments, and it is crucial to work closely with a healthcare provider to find what works best for them. With proper management, many individuals with dysautonomia can lead fulfilling and comfortable lives.

dysautonomia life expentancy

Dysautonomia is a complex disorder

that affects the autonomic nervous system, which is responsible for regulating the body's involuntary functions. This includes things like heart rate, blood pressure, digestion, and temperature control. Dysautonomia can have a significant impact on an individual's quality of life, and one of the most pressing concerns for those living with this condition is their life expectancy. Unfortunately, there is no straightforward answer to the question of life expectancy for those with dysautonomia. This is because dysautonomia encompasses a wide range of conditions, each with its own unique characteristics and potential complications. Therefore, understanding the life expectancy for a person with dysautonomia depends on several factors, including the specific type of dysautonomia, its severity, the age of onset, and any underlying medical conditions. The first thing to understand is that dysautonomia is not a single condition, but a group of disorders that affect the autonomic nervous system. Some of the most common types of dysautonomia include postural orthostatic tachycardia syndrome (POTS), neurocardiogenic syncope (NCS), and pure autonomic failure (PAF). Each of these conditions has its own set of symptoms and potential complications, which can vary significantly from person to person. Therefore, the life expectancy for a person with dysautonomia depends on which of these conditions they have been diagnosed with and how it affects their body. In general, the earlier the onset of dysautonomia, the more severe the symptoms tend to be. This is especially true for conditions like POTS and NCS, which typically affect adolescents and young adults. In contrast, PAF is more commonly seen in older adults and tends to progress more slowly. Therefore, the age at which dysautonomia develops can have a significant impact on a person's life expectancy. Additionally, the severity of dysautonomia can also play a role. Some individuals may experience mild symptoms that are easily managed, while others may have a more severe form of the disorder that greatly impacts their daily life. This can also depend on underlying medical conditions, as dysautonomia can be a secondary disorder to other health issues like diabetes, Parkinson's disease, or connective tissue disorders. One of the biggest challenges with dysautonomia is that it is often difficult to diagnose, leading to delays in treatment and management. As a result, some individuals may not receive a proper diagnosis until later in life when their symptoms have become more severe. This can also have an impact on life expectancy, as proper management and treatment of dysautonomia is essential to help prevent potential complications. Another factor that can impact life expectancy is the presence of comorbidities. Dysautonomia is often associated with other medical conditions that can complicate treatment and management. For example, patients with POTS may also suffer from chronic fatigue syndrome, fibromyalgia, or autoimmune disorders. These co-occurring conditions can further affect a person's overall health and increase the risk of complications, which can ultimately impact life expectancy. One of the most concerning complications of dysautonomia is cardiovascular problems. Some forms of dysautonomia can result in abnormal heart rhythms, blood pressure changes, and issues with blood flow to the heart. This can increase the risk of heart disease, heart attack, and stroke, all of which can significantly impact life expectancy. However, proper management and treatment can help reduce these risks and improve a person's overall health. Unfortunately, there is currently no cure for dysautonomia. Therefore, the goal of treatment is to manage symptoms and maintain a good quality of life. This includes lifestyle modifications, such as increasing fluid and salt intake, wearing compression stockings, and avoiding triggers that can worsen symptoms. Medications may also be prescribed to help control specific symptoms, such as beta-blockers for heart rate control or medications to regulate blood pressure.

chapter2

dysautonomia diagnosis

The diagnosis of dysautonomia often begins with a careful and detailed medical history, along with a physical examination by a healthcare professional. The doctor will ask about the patient's symptoms and when they first started, as well as any potential triggers or factors that may worsen or alleviate their symptoms. A thorough physical exam will also be conducted, which may involve measuring vital signs such as blood pressure, heart rate, and breathing rate. The presence of specific physical findings, such as abnormal sweating or changes in skin color, may also be noted as they can indicate autonomic dysfunction. The next step in the diagnostic process is the use of specialized tests and assessments to evaluate the function of the autonomic nervous system. These tests may vary depending on the symptoms and medical history of the patient, but some of the most commonly used methods include cardiovascular reflex tests, tilt table testing, sweat tests, and thermoregulatory testing. Cardiovascular reflex testing involves measuring the body's response to certain stimuli that normally cause changes in heart rate and blood pressure. This test can provide information on how well the ANS is functioning, as well as any abnormalities or dysfunctions. The tilt table test, on the other hand, is used to diagnose orthostatic intolerance (OI), a common form of dysautonomia. This test involves placing the patient on a table that is tilted to an upright position, mimicking the effect of standing up. Changes in heart rate and blood pressure are closely monitored during this test, and any significant changes may indicate ANS dysfunction. Sweat testing is another important diagnostic method for dysautonomia, as changes in sweating patterns can be a significant indicator of autonomic dysfunction. This test involves applying an irritant substance, such as acetylcholine, to the skin and measuring the body's response. A decreased response or absence of sweating in certain areas may indicate ANS impairment. Similarly, thermoregulatory testing involves changing the environmental temperature to assess the body's ability to maintain its core body temperature. A dysautonomic response may indicate dysfunctions in the ANS that regulate thermoregulation. Apart from these specialized tests, other diagnostic procedures may also be used to rule out other conditions and identify other possible contributing factors. For example, blood tests may be conducted to rule out any underlying medical conditions such as diabetes or thyroid disorders that may be causing symptoms similar to dysautonomia. Additionally, imaging tests, such as MRI or CT scans, may be ordered to evaluate the structure of the brain and spinal cord, where the ANS is located. Electrocardiograms

(ECG) may also be performed to measure the electrical activity of the heart and identify any potential heart abnormalities. It is worth noting that the diagnostic process for dysautonomia can be lengthy and may require multiple tests and evaluations. This is because symptoms of dysautonomia can be nonspecific and similar to those of other conditions, making it important to rule out other potential causes. Additionally, dysautonomia can affect different parts of the ANS, causing varying symptoms and complications. As a result, a comprehensive and individualized approach is necessary for accurate diagnosis and treatment. Apart from physical and medical tests, patient-reported outcomes also play a crucial role in the diagnostic process for dysautonomia. Patients may be asked to keep a record of their symptoms, their severity, and any potential triggers for a certain period. This diary can help healthcare professionals get a better understanding of the patient's condition, monitor the effectiveness of treatments, and identify patterns or fluctuations in symptoms. Another important aspect of the diagnostic process is the involvement of a multidisciplinary team of healthcare professionals. Dysautonomia is a complex disorder that can impact various bodily functions, which requires the expertise and collaboration of different medical specialists. Depending on the type and severity of dysautonomia, a patient may need to see a neurologist, cardiologist, gastroenterologist, or other specialists to manage their condition effectively

chapter3

dysautonomia nhs

Dysautonomia is a relatively rare condition, affecting approximately one in every 3,000 people in the UK (1). However, due to the wide range of symptoms it presents, it is often misdiagnosed or underdiagnosed. The most common types of dysautonomia include postural orthostatic tachycardia syndrome (POTS), neurocardiogenic syncope, and multiple system atrophy (MSA). These conditions can occur as primary disorders or as secondary to other medical conditions, such as diabetes, Parkinson's disease, or Ehlers-Danlos syndrome. The symptoms of dysautonomia are often variable and unpredictable, making it a challenging condition to live with. People with dysautonomia can experience symptoms in any part of the body regulated by the ANS, making it a multi-system disorder. Common symptoms include lightheadedness, dizziness, fainting, fatigue, brain fog, headaches, heart palpitations, nausea, sweating abnormalities, and gastrointestinal issues. These symptoms can range in severity and frequency, making it difficult for individuals to carry out their daily activities, impacting their physical, emotional, and social well-being. Due to the wide range of symptoms associated with dysautonomia, diagnosis and management require a multidisciplinary approach involving various healthcare professionals, including neurologists, cardiologists, gastroenterologists, and physiotherapists. The NHS plays a crucial role in providing these services to individuals with dysautonomia. The diagnosis process typically involves a detailed medical history and physical examination, as well as specialized tests to assess ANS function, such as tilt-table testing, cardiac autonomic reflex testing, and sudomotor testing. These tests help in identifying the subtype of dysautonomia and developing an appropriate treatment plan. One of the main aims of treatment for dysautonomia is to improve an individual's quality of life by managing their symptoms. As the condition is chronic, management strategies focus on symptom relief and preventing complications. There is no single universal treatment for dysautonomia, and treatment may vary depending on the subtype and severity of symptoms. Lifestyle modifications, such as increasing fluid and salt intake, regular exercise, and avoiding triggers, can help in managing symptoms. Medications are also prescribed to manage specific symptoms, such as beta-blockers for tachycardia, anti-nausea medications, and midodrine for low blood pressure. In cases where dysautonomia is secondary to another medical condition, managing that underlying condition is crucial in improving ANS function. For example, treating diabetes effectively can improve symptoms in people with diabetic dysautonomia. In severe cases, individuals may require hospital admission for intravenous fluids or medications to manage symptoms or in-patient rehabilitation programs. As symptoms can fluctuate, individuals with dysautonomia require long-term monitoring and follow-ups with their healthcare team to adjust their treatment plans as needed. The NHS plays a vital role in providing access to specialized tests and medications for individuals with dysautonomia. However, as this is a rare condition, many people may have to travel long distances to access these services, adding to the already challenging nature of living with dysautonomia. In recent years, there have been efforts to improve awareness and understanding of dysautonomia among healthcare professionals to ensure timely and accurate diagnosis and treatment. The establishment of specialist dysautonomia clinics in major cities has also helped in providing better access to care for those affected by this condition. In addition to medical treatment, the NHS also offers support to individuals with dysautonomia through various resources. These include patient support groups, online forums, and educational materials to help individuals understand and manage their condition better. The NHS also provides access to specialist allied healthcare professionals, such as occupational therapists and physiotherapists, who can help individuals manage their symptoms and improve their daily functioning. These resources are crucial in providing emotional and practical support to people with dysautonomia, many of whom may experience emotional distress due to the impact of the condition on their lives.

chapter4

dysautonomia signs

The most common and often first noticed sign of dysautonomia is dizziness or lightheadedness. This is due to the autonomic nervous system's inability to effectively regulate blood pressure, resulting in a drop in blood pressure when changing positions, such as standing up from a seated or lying position. This can also lead to feelings of weakness, fatigue, and even fainting. Many individuals with dysautonomia may also experience brain fog and difficulty concentrating, which can impact their daily activities and overall quality of life. Another common sign of dysautonomia is heart palpitations or a racing heart. This occurs when the autonomic nervous system fails to regulate heart rate, leading to a sudden increase in heart rate even during times of rest or low physical activity. This can be a very distressing symptom for those with dysautonomia, as it can create a sense of panic and anxiety. Some individuals may also experience chest pain or shortness of breath during episodes of elevated heart rate. Dysautonomia can also affect digestion, causing a wide range of symptoms such as nausea, bloating, constipation, and diarrhea. This is due to the autonomic nervous system's role in regulating digestive functions, such as stomach emptying and bowel movements. Many individuals may also experience difficulty swallowing or a feeling of food getting stuck in their throat, known as dysphagia. These digestive symptoms can greatly impact daily life and may require dietary changes and medications to manage. In addition to these common symptoms, there are also less talked about signs of dysautonomia that individuals may experience. One of these is temperature intolerance, where individuals may have difficulty regulating their body temperature, resulting in fluctuations between feeling too hot or too cold. Others may also experience excessive sweating or an inability to sweat, leading to potential heatstroke or heat exhaustion. This can be particularly problematic during hot weather or when participating in physical activities. Other signs of dysautonomia may include changes in vision, such as blurred or double vision, headaches, and a general feeling of malaise and unease. Many individuals may also have trouble sleeping, often due to the discomfort caused by their symptoms or the presence of a comorbid condition known as Ehlers-Danlos Syndrome (EDS), which is commonly associated with dysautonomia. It is important to note that the signs and symptoms of dysautonomia can vary greatly from person to person. Some individuals may experience only a few of these symptoms, while others may have a combination of several. Additionally, the severity of symptoms can also fluctuate, with some individuals experiencing milder symptoms while others have more debilitating ones.

While dysautonomia can be a challenging condition to manage, there are several treatment options available to help alleviate symptoms and improve quality of life. These may include lifestyle changes such as increased water and salt intake, regular exercise, and a healthy diet. Some individuals may also benefit from medications that help regulate blood pressure and heart rate. One of the most difficult aspects of dysautonomia is the lack of awareness and understanding of the condition. Many individuals may struggle to receive a proper diagnosis as the symptoms can be vague and difficult to pinpoint. This can lead to a prolonged period of uncertainty and frustration, impacting a person's mental health and well-being. Therefore, awareness and education about dysautonomia are crucial.

The end